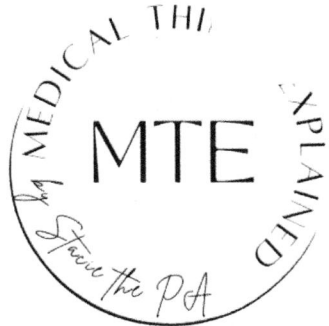

Pneumonia 101: A Patient's Complete Guide to Symptoms, Treatments, and Prevention.

By Stacie the PA

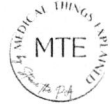

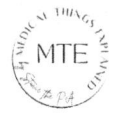

Acknowledgments

I would like to extend my heartfelt gratitude to the teachers, professors, nurses, doctors, physician assistants, nurse practitioners, anesthesiologists, nurse anesthetists, midwives, pharmacists, social workers, technicians, therapists, administrators, and countless other healthcare professionals with whom I have had the privilege of working over the past 20 years.

Your dedication, expertise, and mentorship have not only deepened my knowledge but also inspired the creation of these resources. Thank you for sharing your insights, your time, and your unwavering commitment to patient care. Your guidance has been invaluable to my professional journey, and it is because of each of you that these books have come to life.

This work is a tribute to the profound impact you all have on healthcare and the lives you touch every day.

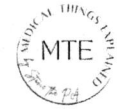

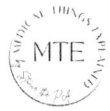

Table of Contents

SECTION 1	**8**
Common Symptoms of Pneumonia	12
SECTION 2	**16**
Glossary of Terms: Related to Pneumonia and Respiratory Care	17
Section 3	**22**
What can you do to reduce your risk of getting pneumonia?	33
What do I do if I think I have pneumonia or the beginning of it?	39
SECTION 5	**44**
How is Pneumonia Diagnosed?	45
Treatments for Pneumonia	47
1. Intubation and Mechanical Ventilation	51
2. Pleural Drainage (Thoracentesis)	53
3. Bronchoscopy	55
4. Surgical Drainage or Decortication	57
SECTION 6	**64**
What is the recovery time after the pneumonia?	65
Factors Affecting Recovery for All Types of Pneumonia	69
What is Pulmonary Rehab? Is Physical therapy needed?	71
What is Mindfulness?	77
How do you do those exercises to reduce anxiety?	77
SECTION 7	**84**
How Pneumonia Affects Spouses and Family Members	85
Understanding the Emotional Impact on Loved Ones	87
How Families Can Cope with the Emotional Impact of Pneumonia	88
How does an illness like pneumonia affect intimacy and self esteem?	90
Summary	94
SECTION 8	**96**
Resources and References	97
SECTION 9	**98**
Personal Medical Summary:	99

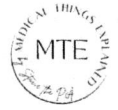

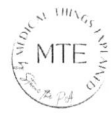

Introduction

Welcome to this patient education workbook on pneumonia! This resource is designed to provide you with essential information about pneumonia, helping you understand the condition, its causes, symptoms, treatment options, and preventive measures. By gaining a deeper understanding of pneumonia, you will be better equipped to take an active role in your health care and recovery.

Purpose of the Workbook

The primary purpose of this workbook is to educate individuals who may not have a medical background about pneumonia. It aims to simplify complex medical information, making it accessible and understandable. Whether you or a loved one is facing pneumonia, this workbook will guide you through important concepts, empowering you to make informed decisions about your health.

Importance of Understanding Pneumonia

Understanding pneumonia is crucial for several reasons. First, it helps you recognize the symptoms early, which can lead to timely medical intervention. Second, knowledge of the causes and risk factors can help you take proactive steps to reduce your chances of developing pneumonia. Lastly, understanding treatment options and recovery processes can alleviate anxiety and foster a sense of control during your health journey.

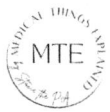

How to Use This Workbook

This workbook is structured to provide information in a clear and straightforward manner. You will find various sections covering different aspects of pneumonia, including its causes, symptoms, diagnosis, treatment, and prevention. Each section includes simple explanations, helpful tips, and questions you may have. Feel free to read through the entire workbook or refer to specific sections as needed. It is also a great idea to keep this workbook handy when discussing your condition with your healthcare provider.

By the end of this workbook, you will have a solid understanding of pneumonia and the tools necessary to manage your health effectively. Let's get started!

SECTION 1

Understanding Pneumonia

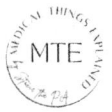

Basic Definitions

Pneumonia is an infection that affects your lungs, which are the sponge-like organs in your chest that help you breathe. Imagine your lungs are like two spongy balloons. When you breathe in, they fill up with air, allowing oxygen to enter your body. When you have pneumonia, it's like those balloons cannot fully inflate because there is sticky goo (infection) in some spots, instead of air. This goo makes it hard for your lungs to inflate all the way.

Pneumonia can be caused by different germs, such as bacteria, viruses, or fungi. These germs can enter your lungs when you breathe, especially if someone nearby is sick. When the germs get into your lungs, they can cause inflammation, which is like a traffic jam in your airways. This makes it difficult for air to flow in and out, leading to symptoms like coughing, fever, and trouble breathing.

In summary, pneumonia is when your lungs become infected and can't do their job as well as they should, making it hard for you to breathe.

Some risk factors can increase the likelihood of developing pneumonia.

According to the Centers for Disease Control and Prevention (CDC), the following groups of people are at a higher risk:

1. **Age:** Young children (especially those under age 2) and older adults (especially those 65 and older) are more susceptible to pneumonia. Their immune systems may not be as robust, making it harder to fight off infections.

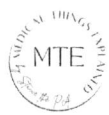

2. **Chronic Health Conditions:** Individuals with chronic diseases such as asthma, chronic obstructive pulmonary disease (COPD), diabetes, or heart disease are at greater risk. These conditions can weaken the immune system or reduce lung function.

3. **Smoking:** Smoking damages the lungs and decreases their ability to fight off infections, making smokers more vulnerable to pneumonia.

4. **Weakened Immune System:** People with weakened immune systems, whether due to conditions like HIV/AIDS, cancer, or immunosuppressive medications (such as those used after organ transplants), are more likely to develop pneumonia.

5. **Recent Respiratory Infections:** Individuals who have recently had a cold, flu, or other respiratory infections may be at increased risk, as these illnesses can make it easier for pneumonia-causing germs to take hold.

6. **Hospitalization:** Being hospitalized, particularly in intensive care units, increases the risk of pneumonia, especially if a person is on a ventilator or has had surgery.

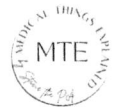

7. **Living in Crowded Conditions:** People living in crowded environments, such as nursing homes, shelters, or military barracks, may be more susceptible due to close contact with others who may be ill.

8. **Alcohol Abuse:** Heavy alcohol consumption can weaken the immune system and impair the body's ability to clear infections, increasing the risk of pneumonia.

For more detailed information, you can visit the CDC's pneumonia page: CDC - Pneumonia.

Pneumonia patients are categorized in 3 major groups:

A. Mild/Non-Hospitalized

Refers to patients who have pneumonia but can manage the condition at home without the need for hospitalization.

B. Severe/Hospitalized

Refers to patients who require hospitalization due to more severe symptoms, such as difficulty breathing or the need for intensive care.

C. High-Risk/Immunocompromised

Refers to patients with weakened immune systems, whether due to chronic illness, medications, or other factors that put them at increased risk for complications from pneumonia.

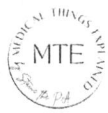

Common Symptoms of Pneumonia

A. **Mild/Non-Hospitalized**: These symptoms are typically seen in patients who are diagnosed with pneumonia but can be managed at home:
- Cough: Often productive, meaning it may produce mucus or phlegm.
- Fever: Mild to moderate fever, sometimes accompanied by chills.
- Shortness of Breath: Difficulty breathing, especially during physical activity.
- Chest Pain: Discomfort or pain in the chest that may worsen with deep breaths or coughing.
- Fatigue: General tiredness or weakness.

B. **Severe/Hospitalized:** Patients requiring hospitalization often present more severe symptoms, reflecting a more serious condition:
- High Fever: Elevated temperatures (often over 101°F or 38.3°C).
- Severe Shortness of Breath: Difficulty breathing at rest, requiring supplemental oxygen or mechanical ventilation.
- Rapid Breathing and Heart Rate: Increased respiratory and heart rates due to the body's stress response.
- Confusion or Altered Mental Status: Especially in older adults, as pneumonia can affect cognition (this is typically reversed after the infection clears)
- Persistent Cough: Often more severe and accompanied by thick, discolored sputum.

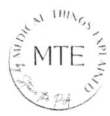

C. **High Risk/Immunocompromised:** Individuals with weakened immune systems (due to conditions like uncontrolled Diabetes, chronic steroid use, those without their spleen, chronic kidney disease, HIV/AIDS, cancer with or without current chemo or radiation treatments, etc) may experience atypical symptoms:
- Subtle Symptoms: Symptoms may not be as pronounced or may develop more slowly, such as a mild cough or low-grade fever.
- Unusual Symptoms: Instead of typical respiratory symptoms, there may be systemic symptoms like night sweats or weight loss.
- Worsening of Underlying Conditions: Symptoms may exacerbate existing health issues rather than presenting as classic pneumonia signs.
- Potential for Atypical Pathogens: The infection may be caused by less common organisms, leading to different symptoms, such as gastrointestinal complaints or skin lesions.

Summary

Recognizing the differences in symptoms based on the setting and immune status is crucial for timely diagnosis and treatment. Outpatients may present with mild to moderate symptoms, while inpatients typically show more severe manifestations, and immunocompromised patients may display atypical or less pronounced symptoms, which can complicate diagnosis and treatment.

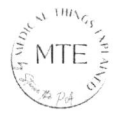

SECTION 2

Glossary of Terms

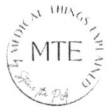

Glossary of Terms: Related to Pneumonia and Respiratory Care

Antibiotics
Medications used to treat bacterial infections. If pneumonia is caused by bacteria, antibiotics may be prescribed to help fight the infection.

Arterial Blood Gas (ABG)
A blood test that measures the oxygen and carbon dioxide levels in your blood to see how well your lungs are working.

Bacteria
Tiny organisms that can cause infections like bacterial pneumonia. Bacteria are one of the most common causes of pneumonia.

Bronchoscopy
A medical procedure where a doctor uses a small camera on a tube (called a bronchoscope) to look inside the lungs and airways. It can help diagnose pneumonia or collect samples of mucus.

Chest X-ray (CXR)
A picture of the chest using X-rays to help doctors see your lungs and check for signs of pneumonia or other lung problems.

Chronic Obstructive Pulmonary Disease (COPD)
A long-term lung disease that makes it hard to breathe and can increase the risk of getting pneumonia.

Cyanosis
A bluish color that can appear on the lips, face, or fingers, often caused by low oxygen levels in the blood. It can be a sign that pneumonia is affecting the lungs' ability to deliver oxygen.

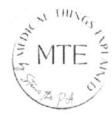

Cough
A common symptom of pneumonia where you may cough up mucus or phlegm from your lungs.

Fever
A higher-than-normal body temperature, which is often a sign that the body is fighting an infection like pneumonia.

Inhalers
Devices used to deliver medication directly into your lungs. Inhalers can help open your airways, making it easier to breathe.

Intensive Care Unit (ICU)
A special hospital unit where seriously ill patients receive advanced care, including breathing support if necessary, such as using a ventilator.

Intubation
A medical procedure where a tube is inserted into the airway to help someone breathe. This is often done if the person is very sick and can't breathe on their own.

Lungs
The organs in your chest that help you breathe. Your lungs have two sides (right and left), and each side has different lobes (sections). The right lung has three lobes, while the left lung has two lobes. Pneumonia can affect one or more lobes of the lungs, making it difficult to breathe.

Oxygen Therapy
Treatment that provides extra oxygen to help you breathe better if your lungs aren't getting enough oxygen on their own due to pneumonia.

PEEP (Positive End-Expiratory Pressure)
A setting on a ventilator that helps keep the airways open by adding pressure to the lungs at the end of exhalation. This can help improve oxygen levels in people with severe pneumonia.

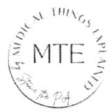

Pneumonia
An infection of the lungs that causes inflammation and difficulty breathing. It can be caused by bacteria, viruses, or fungi.

Pulse Oximeter
A small device that clips to your finger and measures how much oxygen is in your blood. It helps doctors check if your lungs are getting enough oxygen.

Rales/Crackles
The sounds that can be heard when a doctor listens to your lungs with a stethoscope. These crackling sounds often happen when air passes through fluid or mucus in the lungs, which can occur with pneumonia.

Steroids
Medications that reduce inflammation. Sometimes used to help with breathing problems during pneumonia, though they are not always used for everyone.

Ventilator
A machine that helps people breathe when they are unable to breathe on their own. This is often used for very sick patients in the hospital.

Viral Pneumonia
A type of pneumonia caused by a virus, like the flu or COVID-19. It is usually treated differently from bacterial pneumonia.

Wheezing
A high-pitched sound that can occur when breathing, often caused by difficulty breathing. Wheezing may happen if the airways in the lungs are blocked or narrowed, which can happen with pneumonia.

Section 3

Prepare for Office Visit

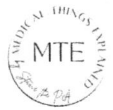

When being evaluated for possible pneumonia, there are several key questions YOU should be prepared to answer. These questions help your medical provider assess the severity of your condition, identify potential causes, and determine the appropriate treatment. Here are some important questions:

1. What are your symptoms?

- Describe any symptoms you're experiencing, such as coughing, fever, chills, shortness of breath, chest pain, fatigue, or confusion.

2. When did your symptoms start?

- Knowing the onset of symptoms helps doctors understand how long the infection may have been developing and how severe it might be.

3. Have you been exposed to anyone with similar symptoms?

- Pneumonia can be contagious, especially if it's caused by a virus or bacteria. Knowing about possible exposure to sick people helps doctors assess risk.

4. Do you have any existing health conditions?

- Chronic conditions like asthma, diabetes, heart disease, COPD, or kidney disease can increase your risk for pneumonia. This also includes autoimmune diseases and conditions that suppress the immune system.

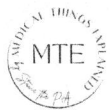

5. Are you currently taking any medications?

- Certain medications, like steroids or immunosuppressants, can increase the risk of infections, including pneumonia. What over the counter medications have you tried since this started? Have they been helpful? Do you already use inhalers or nebulizers?

6. Have you recently had a cold, flu, or other respiratory illness?

- Pneumonia can sometimes develop after a viral infection like the flu or a cold, so it's important to know if you've had any recent respiratory illnesses.

7. Are you a smoker? Do you vape? Are you around second hand smoke frequently?

- Smoking damages the lungs and weakens the body's ability to fight off infections, increasing the risk of pneumonia.

8. Do you have a history of pneumonia or other lung diseases?

- Previous lung conditions, such as pneumonia, tuberculosis, or chronic lung diseases, may increase your risk for developing pneumonia again. Were you ever hospitalized for these issues? Did you need a breathing tube?

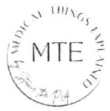

9. Have you been hospitalized recently?

- Recent hospital stays, especially if you've been in an ICU or on a ventilator, increase the risk of hospital-acquired pneumonia.

10. Have you had a pneumonia vaccination?

- There are vaccines available that can help prevent certain types of pneumonia. It's helpful for doctors to know if you've had these vaccines. Where, when, what type, who has those records?

11. Have you noticed any NEW CHANGES in your ability to breathe?

- Difficulty breathing, shortness of breath, or feeling winded with minimal activity can be signs of pneumonia or other lung issues.

12. Do you have a fever or chills?

- Fever is a common symptom of pneumonia. Knowing whether you have a fever, and how high it is, can help doctors determine the severity of the infection. Keep a record of your temperature at home.

13. Do you have any rib, chest, lung pain when breathing or coughing?

- This would be different from your normal pains. Chest pain, especially when taking deep breaths or coughing, can indicate pneumonia or another lung issue like pleuritis (inflammation of the lining of the lungs).

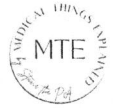

14. Have you been exposed to environmental hazards?

- Exposure to certain environments, like dusty work settings, outdoor pollution, or workshop exposures like silica dust, wood dust, recent spring cleaning and exposure to cleaning chemicals you are not used to, may increase the risk of pneumonia.

15. What is your general health like?

- Knowing if you have a strong immune system or if you're at higher risk (due to age or other factors) helps the doctor assess the urgency of the situation. Are you on oxygen, CPAP overnight?

These questions are part of the initial evaluation and help the healthcare provider understand the potential causes, risk factors, and the seriousness of your symptoms. Being prepared to answer them can make the evaluation process smoother and help the doctor determine the best course of action.

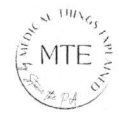

SECTION 4

Lifestyle Changes and Self-Management

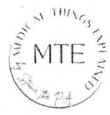

What can you do to reduce your risk of getting pneumonia?

Preventing pneumonia involves adopting lifestyle changes that support overall lung health and strengthen the immune system. Here are some key lifestyle changes that can help reduce the risk of developing pneumonia:

1. Quit Smoking

- Smoking damages the lungs, weakens the immune system, and increases the risk of respiratory infections, including pneumonia. Quitting smoking improves lung function and reduces the likelihood of infections.

2. Practice Good Hygiene

- Regular handwashing with soap and water can help prevent the spread of germs that cause respiratory infections. Use hand sanitizer when soap and water aren't available.
- Cover your mouth and nose with a tissue or your elbow when coughing or sneezing to prevent spreading germs to others.
- Clean and disinfect frequently-touched surfaces, especially during cold and flu season.

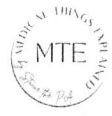

3. Get Vaccinated

- Vaccines are one of the most effective ways to prevent certain types of pneumonia, please discuss these with your medical provider:
    - **Pneumococcal Vaccine**: This vaccine helps protect against pneumonia caused by the *Streptococcus pneumoniae* bacteria.
    - **Flu Vaccine**: Since the flu can lead to pneumonia, getting a yearly flu shot reduces the risk of developing pneumonia as a complication of the flu.
    - **COVID-19 Vaccine**: The COVID-19 virus can cause pneumonia, so vaccination helps reduce the risk of severe respiratory illness and pneumonia.

4. Maintain a Healthy Diet

- Eating a balanced diet rich in fruits, vegetables, whole grains, and lean proteins can strengthen the immune system and support lung health. Nutrients like vitamins A, C, and E, as well as zinc, are particularly important for immune function.
- Drinking plenty of fluids helps keep the respiratory system hydrated and supports the body's ability to clear mucus from the lungs.

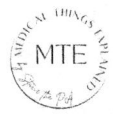

5. Exercise Regularly

- Regular physical activity strengthens the lungs and improves immune function. It also helps prevent chronic conditions like heart disease, COPD, and diabetes, which can increase the risk of pneumonia.
- Aim for at least 150 minutes of moderate-intensity exercise or 75 minutes of vigorous-intensity exercise per week.

6. Avoid Exposure to Respiratory Illnesses

- Stay away from individuals who are sick, especially those with respiratory infections such as the flu or cold.
- If possible, avoid crowded places during peak flu and cold seasons to reduce the risk of catching pneumonia-causing viruses and bacteria.

7. Keep Your Home Clean and Free from Allergens

- Regularly clean your home to reduce dust, mold, and pet dander, which can irritate the lungs and increase the risk of respiratory infections. Using a HEPA filter in your home can help reduce airborne allergens.
- Make sure your home is well-ventilated to prevent the growth of mold, which can cause respiratory issues.

8. Manage Chronic Health Conditions

- Properly manage chronic health conditions like diabetes, asthma, COPD, and heart disease. Keeping these conditions under control can reduce the risk of developing pneumonia.

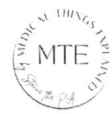

- Take medications as prescribed and attend regular check-ups with your healthcare provider to monitor and manage chronic conditions.

9. Get Enough Sleep

- Adequate sleep (7-9 hours per night for most adults) is crucial for maintaining a strong immune system. Sleep helps the body repair and regenerate, reducing the risk of infections.

10. Stay Hydrated

- Drinking plenty of water helps thin mucus in the lungs, making it easier to expel. It also helps maintain a healthy respiratory system and supports overall immune function.

11. Use a Humidifier

- Keeping the air in your home moist with a humidifier can prevent your airways from becoming dry, which helps reduce irritation in the lungs and airways. This is particularly helpful during colder months when the air is drier.

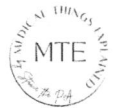

12. Reduce Stress

- Chronic stress can weaken the immune system, making it harder for the body to fight off infections. Practice stress-reducing techniques such as yoga, meditation, deep breathing, or other relaxation methods.

By adopting these lifestyle changes, you can help prevent pneumonia and support your overall lung and immune health. These habits are especially important for individuals who are at higher risk for pneumonia, including the elderly, those with chronic health conditions, and smokers.

The information provided comes from a combination of reputable health sources, including guidance from the **Centers for Disease Control and Prevention (CDC), World Health Organization (WHO)**, and other public health resources that focus on pneumonia prevention and general respiratory health. These organizations offer evidence-based recommendations for preventing pneumonia and maintaining good lung health.

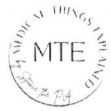

What do I do if I think I have pneumonia or the beginning of it?

If you think you may have pneumonia, it's important to take the right steps for self-management, but always seek medical attention to confirm the diagnosis and receive proper treatment. Here are some things you can do for self-management when you suspect you have pneumonia:

1. Seek Medical Care

- **Consult your medical provider (ask for the first available urgent visit appointment)** as soon as possible if you experience symptoms like persistent cough, fever, difficulty breathing, or chest pain. Pneumonia can be serious, and early treatment is key to recovery.
- If your symptoms worsen, or if you're having trouble breathing, seek emergency medical attention immediately.

2. Follow Your Provider's Instructions

- If diagnosed with pneumonia, take any prescribed medications (like antibiotics or antivirals) exactly as directed. Completing the full course of antibiotics is important to ensure the infection is fully treated.
- If your doctor recommends medications for managing symptoms, like cough suppressants or pain relievers, use them according to their instructions.

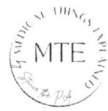

3. Rest and Take It Easy

- Rest is essential to help your body fight the infection and recover. Avoid strenuous activities, and make sure you're getting plenty of sleep to allow your immune system to work efficiently.
- While rest is important, try to get up and move around a bit if you can, as staying completely bed bound can increase the risk of complications, like blood clots or muscle weakness.

4. Stay Hydrated

- Drink plenty of fluids such as water, herbal teas, or broth. Staying hydrated helps loosen mucus in your lungs and keeps your respiratory system hydrated, which can aid in your recovery.

5. Use a Humidifier

- A humidifier can help keep the air moist, which can soothe irritated airways and make it easier to breathe. This can be especially helpful if you're experiencing a dry cough or congestion.

6. Manage Your Fever

- If you have a fever, use over-the-counter fever reducers like acetaminophen (Tylenol) or ibuprofen (Advil, Motrin), but only as recommended by your healthcare provider. Resting, staying cool, and drinking fluids can also help manage fever.

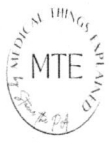

7. Coughing and Deep Breathing Exercises

- **Coughing** helps clear mucus from your lungs, which is important for recovery. Use a tissue or cough into your elbow to prevent spreading germs to others.
- **Deep breathing exercises** can help you expand your lungs and improve airflow. Try breathing in deeply through your nose, holding it for a few seconds, and then exhaling slowly through your mouth.

8. Elevate Your Head While Sleeping

- If you're having trouble breathing or coughing a lot at night, elevate your head with pillows while you sleep to help clear mucus from your lungs and make breathing easier.

9. Avoid Smoking and Secondhand Smoke

- Smoking can irritate your lungs and make it harder to recover from pneumonia. Avoid smoking, and try to stay away from secondhand smoke as much as possible.

10. Nutrition

- Eating a balanced diet with plenty of fruits, vegetables, and proteins helps support your immune system. Nutrients like vitamin C, vitamin D, and zinc play a role in immune function and recovery.

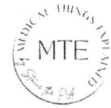

11. Monitor Your Symptoms

- Keep track of your symptoms and note any changes. If you experience worsening symptoms, such as increasing difficulty breathing, chest pain, or confusion, seek medical care immediately.

12. Prevent the Spread of Germs

- Pneumonia can be contagious, especially if it's caused by a virus or bacteria. Wash your hands frequently, cover your mouth when coughing, and avoid close contact with others until you're feeling better.

Red Flags to Watch For:

While self-management is important, there are certain signs that indicate the need for immediate medical attention, including:

- **Severe difficulty breathing** (feeling like you can't catch your breath)
- **Chest pain** that doesn't go away or worsens with deep breathing
- **Confusion or altered mental status**, especially in older adults
- **Cyanosis** (a bluish tint to the lips or skin), which indicates low oxygen levels
- **Persistent high fever** that doesn't respond to fever reducers

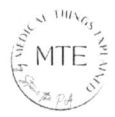

SECTION 5

Diagnosis, Treatments and Interventions.

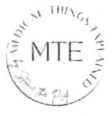

How is Pneumonia Diagnosed?

Pneumonia is diagnosed through a combination of medical history, physical examination, and tests. Depending on the severity and type of pneumonia (mild, severe, or in immunocompromised patients), the medical provider may use different methods to diagnose it.

1. **Medical History and Symptoms:**
   - The medical provider will ask about your symptoms, like coughing, fever, shortness of breath, and chest pain. They will also ask about any recent illnesses, such as a cold or flu, and if you have any chronic health conditions like asthma or heart disease.

2. **Physical Examination:**
   - During the exam, the medical provider will listen to your lungs with a stethoscope. They may hear crackling or wheezing sounds, which can be signs of pneumonia. They may also check your temperature, breathing rate, and oxygen levels.

3. **Chest X-ray (CXR):**
   - A chest X-ray is often used to get a clear picture of your lungs. It helps the medical provider see if there is any fluid or infection in the lungs that would suggest pneumonia.

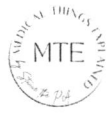

4. **Blood Tests:**
    - Blood tests can help detect signs of infection. Medical providers may check for an increased white blood cell count or take blood cultures to see if bacteria or other germs are causing the infection

5. **Sputum Test:**
    - If you have a cough, the medical provider might ask for a sample of the mucus (sputum) you are coughing up. This can help identify the bacteria or virus causing the infection.

6. **Pulse Oximetry:**
    - This is a small device clipped to your finger that measures the oxygen level in your blood. If your oxygen levels are low, it can indicate that your lungs aren't working as well as they should.

7. **Additional Tests for Severe or Immunocompromised Patients:**
    - If pneumonia is suspected to be more severe, or if the patient has a weakened immune system, medical providers may perform additional tests like a CT scan or a bronchoscopy (a test where a tube is used to view the inside of the lungs).

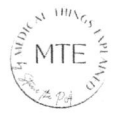

Treatments for Pneumonia

Treatment for pneumonia depends on the type, severity, and whether the patient has other health issues. Here's an overview of general treatment options:

A. Mild Pneumonia (Non-Hospitalized/Outpatient):
- **Antibiotics or Antivirals**: If the pneumonia is caused by bacteria, antibiotics are prescribed. If it's caused by a virus, antiviral medications may be used. The type of medication depends on the specific germ causing the infection.
- **Rest**: Getting plenty of rest is important for helping your body fight the infection and heal.
- **Fluids**: Drinking plenty of fluids helps keep you hydrated, loosen mucus, and make it easier to breathe.
- **Pain and Fever Relief**: Over-the-counter medications like acetaminophen (Tylenol) or ibuprofen (Advil) can help reduce fever and chest pain.

B. For Severe Pneumonia (Hospitalized/Inpatient):
- **IV Antibiotics or Antivirals**: Patients with severe pneumonia often need stronger medications given through an IV (into a vein) to quickly fight the infection.
- **Oxygen Therapy**: If pneumonia is making it hard to breathe, supplemental oxygen can help increase the amount of oxygen in the blood and make breathing easier.

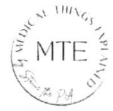

- **Ventilator**: In very severe cases, when breathing is extremely difficult, a ventilator may be used to help the patient breathe.
- **Fluid Management**: In some cases, patients may need IV fluids to maintain hydration or manage low blood pressure.

C. For Immunocompromised Patients (Weakened Immune System):

- **Targeted Treatment**: Patients with a weakened immune system may require specific treatments based on the type of infection. Medical providers might use a combination of antibiotics, antifungals, or antivirals, depending on the cause of pneumonia.
- **Close Monitoring**: Because their immune systems are weaker, immunocompromised patients need closer monitoring, often in the hospital, to ensure that any complications are caught early.
- **Supportive Care**: Immunocompromised patients may need additional support, such as oxygen therapy or ventilator assistance, if their pneumonia affects their ability to breathe.

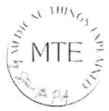

Summary

Pneumonia is diagnosed through a combination of symptom review, physical exams, and tests like chest X-rays and blood tests. The treatment depends on how severe the pneumonia is and whether the patient has other health issues. Mild pneumonia can often be treated at home with antibiotics, rest, and fluids, while severe pneumonia may require hospitalization with stronger medications and breathing support. For immunocompromised patients, special care is needed to prevent complications and provide appropriate treatment.

The information provided is based on general guidelines and recommendations from well-known health organizations, such as:

Centers for Disease Control and Prevention (CDC): The CDC offers detailed information on the diagnosis, treatment, and prevention of pneumonia. Their guidelines include information for both bacterial and viral pneumonia, as well as specific considerations for severe and immunocompromised patients. CDC - Pneumonia

American Lung Association (ALA): The ALA provides guidelines on pneumonia symptoms, diagnosis, and treatment, with specific emphasis on prevention strategies such as vaccination and smoking cessation. American Lung Association - Pneumonia

National Institutes of Health (NIH): The NIH provides extensive resources on respiratory health, including pneumonia diagnosis, treatment options, and care for vulnerable populations like those with weakened immune systems. NIH - Pneumonia

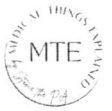

When pneumonia is more serious, what are the procedures that may be done?

There are some invasive treatments used for the treatment of pneumonia, particularly in severe cases or when complications arise. These treatments are typically used when the pneumonia is not responding to standard treatments, or when the patient has a weakened immune system or other complicating factors. Here are a few examples of invasive treatments:

1. Intubation and Mechanical Ventilation

- **When Used**: For patients with severe pneumonia who are unable to breathe on their own or who have dangerously low oxygen levels, intubation may be required. A tube is inserted into the airway (trachea) to help with breathing, and a ventilator (a machine) may be used to assist with breathing or fully take over the breathing process.
- **Purpose**: This is done to maintain oxygen levels in the blood and prevent respiratory failure. It is usually done in critical care settings, such as an ICU.

More questions about this:

When someone is intubated and put on a ventilator, they are usually not aware of the tube being placed or the machine breathing for them because they are given medications to help them relax or sleep. This is done to make the procedure more comfortable and to ensure the person doesn't feel pain or discomfort during the process. Here's a breakdown of what typically happens:

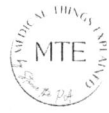

Do They Know the Tube Is Being Placed?

No. When a person is intubated, they are usually given a medication to make them unconscious or very relaxed (called anesthesia or sedatives). This helps the person not feel or remember the tube being inserted into their airway.

Do They Feel Pain?

No. The procedure of inserting the tube is done while the person is sedated, so they don't feel pain during the intubation. However, once the tube is in place and they wake up, they may feel some discomfort in their throat or chest, like soreness or a feeling of pressure. Medical providers may give them pain-relieving medications to help with this discomfort.

Are They Scared?

Not while sedated. Since the person is unconscious or heavily sedated during the intubation, they typically don't experience fear during the procedure. In most cases, if someone needs the breathing machine, they are not aware enough to be fearful, and or they are sedated to make this process less traumatic for them. Once they wake up, they might feel anxious, confused, or scared, especially if they don't fully understand why they're on a ventilator or how long they will need it. This is common, and the healthcare team works to comfort the person and explain what is happening.

In summary, while the person is being intubated and on a ventilator, they typically don't feel pain or fear because they are sedated. Afterward, they might experience some discomfort or anxiety, but this can be managed with pain relief and reassurance from the medical team.

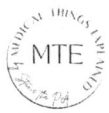

2. Pleural Drainage (Thoracentesis)

- **When Used**: If pneumonia causes fluid to build up in the pleural space (the area between the lungs and chest wall), this is known as a pleural effusion. If the fluid is infected (parapneumonic effusion or empyema), it may need to be drained.
- **Purpose**: A needle or small tube is inserted into the chest to remove the fluid. This helps reduce pressure on the lungs and allows them to expand more easily, making breathing less difficult. In some cases, the drainage tube may be left in place for several days.

More questions about this:

When someone undergoes pleural drainage (also known as thoracentesis), the procedure is usually done to remove excess fluid from around the lungs, which can help with breathing. Here's what typically happens:

Do They Know the Procedure Is Happening?

Yes, the person is usually awake during a thoracentesis, but they are given a local anesthetic (numbing medicine) to numb the area where the needle or tube will be inserted. This means they shouldn't feel pain in the area being treated, though they may feel some pressure or a slight discomfort.

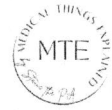

Do They Feel Pain?

Not typically during the procedure. The local anesthetic numbs the skin and the tissue where the needle or tube is inserted, so the person doesn't feel pain in that specific area. However, they might feel some pressure as the fluid is being removed. After the procedure, there could be some soreness or mild discomfort in the area where the needle or tube was inserted, but this can usually be managed with pain relief if needed.

Are They Scared?

It depends. Some people may feel nervous or anxious because they are awake during the procedure and might be unsure about what's happening. It's natural to feel worried when you're having a procedure done, especially one involving your lungs. The medical team will usually explain the procedure clearly and try to make the person feel as comfortable and calm as possible. They may also give medication to help relax the person if needed.

In summary, while a pleural drainage (thoracentesis) is happening, the person typically doesn't feel pain due to the numbing medicine, but they may feel some pressure. Afterward, there may be some soreness or discomfort in the area, but it can usually be treated. The person might feel anxious or scared, but the medical providers will work to help reassure and comfort them throughout the procedure.

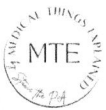

3. Bronchoscopy

- **When Used**: In cases where there is difficulty in clearing mucus or if the pneumonia is suspected to be caused by a blockage (e.g., foreign objects or tumors), a **bronchoscopy** may be performed. This procedure is also helpful when doctors need to collect sputum samples from deep within the lungs.
- **Purpose**: A bronchoscope (a thin, flexible tube with a camera) is inserted through the mouth or nose and into the lungs. It allows the medical provider to visualize the airways, remove obstructions, and take samples for testing. It is often used in severe or complicated pneumonia cases, such as in immunocompromised patients.

More information about this:

When someone undergoes a bronchoscopy, the procedure is used to look inside the lungs and airways, often to collect samples or check for any issues like infection, blockages, or tumors. Here's what typically happens:

Do They Know the Procedure Is Happening?

It depends on the type of sedation. In most cases, the person is awake but given a sedative or a mild anesthetic to help them relax and make the procedure more comfortable. The sedative might make them feel sleepy or a little dizzy, but they are generally aware of what's happening during the bronchoscopy. If a deeper level of sedation is used (or general anesthesia in more complex cases), the person may be asleep and unaware of the procedure.

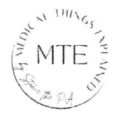

Do They Feel Pain?

No, there should be no pain. A bronchoscopy involves inserting a small, flexible tube (the bronchoscope) into the airways through the nose or mouth, and the area where the tube enters is numbed with a local anesthetic. The numbing medicine helps prevent pain. The person may feel some discomfort, like a sensation of pressure, coughing, or gagging, as the tube is moved into the lungs. However, these sensations shouldn't be painful due to the sedatives and numbing medicine. After the procedure, there might be some mild soreness or irritation in the throat, which can usually be treated with over-the-counter pain relief if needed.

Are They Scared?

It's normal to feel anxious. Many people might feel nervous or worried about having a bronchoscopy because it involves the airways and might seem a little invasive. However, medical providers explain the procedure in advance and reassure the person. Sedation is often used to help make the experience more comfortable, and after the procedure, the person may feel groggy or disoriented for a short time, which can also add to anxiety. It's normal to feel uneasy, but medical providers are trained to support the person and help them stay calm throughout.

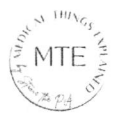

In summary, during a bronchoscopy, the person is usually aware of the procedure but may be relaxed or sedated to reduce discomfort. They generally don't feel pain because the area is numbed, but they might feel some pressure, coughing, or mild discomfort. Afterward, there could be a sore throat or irritation, but this is usually temporary. Some people might feel nervous or anxious, but the medical team will work to make the process as comfortable and reassuring as possible.

4. Surgical Drainage or Decortication

- **When Used**: For severe cases of pneumonia complicated by a large pleural effusion or abscess (a pocket of infected fluid in the lung), surgery may be required to remove the infected tissue or to drain the abscess.
- **Purpose**: If the infection doesn't respond to antibiotics and other treatments, surgical intervention may be necessary to remove the infected material and prevent further spread of the infection.

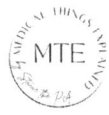

This one is more complicated, more information here:

Decortication, also known as **pleural decortication**, is a surgical procedure used to remove the thickened layer of tissue (called the "pleural peel") that surrounds the lungs in certain severe cases of pneumonia, especially when an infection has caused the pleura (the lining around the lungs) to become inflamed and thickened. This procedure is often done when a patient has **empyema** (a collection of pus in the pleural space) or a **pleural effusion** (fluid buildup), which can occur as a complication of pneumonia. The goal of the surgery is to remove the thickened pleural tissue and improve lung function, which is otherwise restricted due to the tissue's build-up.

Procedure Overview:

Surgical Name: Pleural Decortication.

When It's Performed: It is often performed when pneumonia leads to complications, such as the development of a pleural effusion (fluid buildup between the lungs and chest wall) or empyema (pus in the pleural space). These conditions can cause difficulty breathing and prevent the lungs from fully expanding.

The Surgery: The procedure is typically performed by a **thoracic surgeon**, who is a specialist in surgeries of the chest, including the lungs and heart. The surgery is done in the operating room under general anesthesia, which means the patient will be asleep and pain-free during the procedure. During the surgery, the surgeon makes an incision in the chest to access the lungs and pleura. The thickened or infected tissue is carefully removed to allow the lung to expand properly and

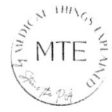

restore normal breathing. This procedure may also involve draining any remaining pus or fluid in the pleural space.

Recovery: After the surgery, patients typically need to stay in the hospital for monitoring and recovery. Recovery may include pain management, chest tube drainage, and physical therapy to help with lung function.

Why It's Done:

Persistent or Severe Infection: Decortication is often necessary when the infection (such as empyema) is not responding to antibiotics, and the thickened pleura is restricting lung function.

Improved Lung Function: The procedure helps to free the lungs from the pleural layers that prevent them from fully expanding, improving breathing and oxygen intake.

5. Extracorporeal Membrane Oxygenation (ECMO)

- **When Used**: This is used in very severe cases of pneumonia, particularly when a patient's lungs are no longer able to provide enough oxygen to the body or remove enough carbon dioxide.
- **Purpose**: ECMO is a machine that pumps and oxygenates a patient's blood outside of the body, allowing the lungs to rest and heal while still providing oxygen to the body. It is a highly specialized and invasive treatment used as a last resort in critical care situations.

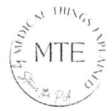

This is quite rare, but still used in some cases. Here is more info:

Extracorporeal Membrane Oxygenation (ECMO) is a highly specialized and advanced life-support treatment that is used in **severe cases of respiratory or cardiac failure**, including when pneumonia leads to **severe respiratory failure**. It provides oxygen to the blood and helps remove carbon dioxide when the lungs or heart can no longer perform these functions adequately. Here's a breakdown of how ECMO is used, who has access to it, and what the recovery prospects are:

How Often Is ECMO Used?

Rarely: ECMO is generally a last-resort treatment and is not commonly used in most cases of pneumonia. It is typically reserved for **extremely severe cases** when other treatment options, such as mechanical ventilation or medication, have not been effective, or when the patient's lungs are unable to provide sufficient oxygen to the body.

When It's Needed: ECMO may be considered for patients who are facing **acute respiratory distress syndrome (ARDS)** or **severe pneumonia** that causes life-threatening breathing problems. It's also used in patients who are critically ill due to heart failure or a combination of both heart and lung failure.

Do Hospitals Need Special Equipment for ECMO?

Yes, ECMO machines require specialized facilities: ECMO is a complex and resource-intensive procedure, so it is generally available only in **large, specialized hospitals** or **academic medical centers**. These hospitals must have the necessary equipment and trained medical teams, including **intensive care**

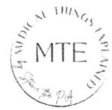

specialists and **cardiothoracic surgeons**, who are experienced in managing ECMO patients.

Dedicated ECMO teams: The care provided to patients on ECMO requires a specialized team that is available 24/7 to monitor and manage the machine, the patient's oxygen levels, and other vital functions.

Likelihood of Recovery with ECMO

Recovery rates vary: ECMO is a life-saving intervention, but it is not a guarantee of recovery. The likelihood of recovery depends on several factors, including the patient's underlying health, the severity of the disease, the cause of the respiratory failure, and how quickly ECMO is initiated.

Higher survival rates with early intervention: Studies suggest that the sooner ECMO is used, the better the chances for recovery. Patients who receive ECMO treatment early in the course of severe respiratory failure or pneumonia may have better outcomes than those who are treated later when organ failure is more advanced.

Variable outcomes: The overall survival rate for ECMO patients depends on the underlying condition. For instance:

Pneumonia-related ECMO: The likelihood of survival with ECMO for pneumonia can vary, with reports suggesting that around 50-60% of patients with severe pneumonia who undergo ECMO survive. However, the recovery rate also depends on how well the lungs heal after ECMO support and whether other organs (like the kidneys or heart) are affected.

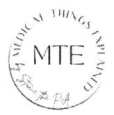

Heart or lung failure: The recovery rates for ECMO also depend on the severity of heart or lung failure and the patient's general health, age, and any other comorbid conditions.

Long-Term Recovery

Recovery after ECMO: Even if a patient survives ECMO, recovery can be slow. Many patients require **physical therapy**, **respiratory rehabilitation**, and sometimes **psychological support** after ECMO because it is a physically and emotionally draining process. Some patients may experience long-term effects, such as muscle weakness or neurological effects from the time spent on the machine.

Some patients may recover completely, especially if ECMO was used for a reversible cause (like severe pneumonia) and if the treatment was timely. Others may have long-term complications due to the severity of their illness.

Summary

ECMO is used in severe, life-threatening cases of respiratory failure, including in patients with pneumonia, but it is not common and is only used in **specialized hospitals** with the necessary equipment and expertise.

The likelihood of recovery varies based on the patient's condition and how early ECMO is applied, but **survival rates** are generally higher when ECMO is initiated early and the underlying condition is treatable.

Recovery is possible, but it may take time and require ongoing care, including rehabilitation.

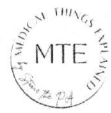

Sources:

- **American Heart Association (AHA)**: Provides resources on ECMO use in cardiac and respiratory failure. AHA - ECMO
- **National Institutes of Health (NIH)**: Offers research and data on ECMO use and recovery rates in critically ill patients. NIH - ECMO

SECTION 6

Recovery and Rehabilitation

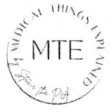

What is the recovery time after the pneumonia?

The typical recovery time and process for pneumonia can vary depending on the type of pneumonia, the severity of the illness, and the patient's overall health.

A. Mild Pneumonia (Non-Hospitalized / Outpatient Pneumonia)

Generally, 1 to 3 weeks for most healthy adults.

Symptoms may start to improve after a few days of treatment, but complete recovery can take a few weeks.

Recovery Process:

Antibiotics or antivirals: If the pneumonia is bacterial, antibiotics will help clear the infection. If it's viral, antiviral medications may be prescribed. In many cases, mild pneumonia is treated successfully at home with these medications.

Rest and hydration: Adequate rest, staying hydrated, and eating a nutritious diet are important for the recovery process.

Symptom relief: Over-the-counter medications, like acetaminophen or ibuprofen, can help relieve pain and reduce fever. Coughing may persist for several weeks, even after the infection is gone.

Follow-up care: Some people may need follow-up visits with their healthcare provider to ensure that the infection has cleared and that they are recovering fully.

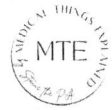

Recovery Outlook:

- Most healthy individuals make a full recovery from mild pneumonia without long-term effects, although they may feel fatigued for a while after the acute symptoms resolve.
- **Coughing** can linger for a few weeks as the lungs heal and clear the remaining mucus.

B. Severe Pneumonia (Hospitalized Pneumonia)

Recovery Time:

> **Hospitalization recovery** may take anywhere from **a few days to several weeks**, depending on the severity of the pneumonia and whether complications (like pleural effusion or sepsis) arise.
>
> After discharge, full recovery can take **several weeks to months**, and some patients may need **rehabilitation** or physical therapy.

Recovery Process:

> **Antibiotics or IV antivirals**: Severe pneumonia often requires intravenous (IV) antibiotics or antivirals. In some cases, patients are treated with oxygen therapy, and mechanical ventilation may be necessary if they are unable to breathe on their own.
>
> **Supportive care**: This may include fluids to prevent dehydration, pain management, and respiratory support (such as oxygen or a ventilator).

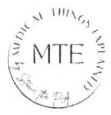

Hospital rehabilitation: If the pneumonia caused long-term effects, physical therapy or pulmonary rehabilitation might be needed to help the patient regain strength and lung function.

Recovery Outlook:

People with severe pneumonia may experience fatigue, muscle weakness, and difficulty breathing for weeks after they leave the hospital.

Follow-up care: Regular follow-up appointments are essential to ensure that the lungs are healing properly and that there are no ongoing complications.

---

3. Immunocompromised Pneumonia (Pneumonia in Weakened Immune Systems)

Recovery Time:

Varies widely depending on the underlying condition, the cause of pneumonia, and how well the immune system responds to treatment.

Recovery can take **longer** than for otherwise healthy individuals and may extend from **several weeks to several months**, especially if the immune system is compromised due to conditions like HIV/AIDS, cancer treatments, or organ transplants.

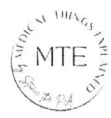

Recovery Process:

Targeted treatment: People with weakened immune systems may require more specialized treatments, including antibiotics, antivirals, or antifungal medications, depending on the type of pneumonia.

Ongoing monitoring: Regular hospital visits may be needed to monitor lung function and other health conditions. These patients are also at higher risk of complications, such as secondary infections.

Respiratory support: Some immunocompromised patients may require additional oxygen therapy or ventilation if their lungs are severely affected.

Recovery Outlook:

The recovery of immunocompromised individuals can be **slower** due to the weakened immune system. They may also experience **relapses** or **complications** during recovery.

Higher risk of complications: Pneumonia in immunocompromised individuals can be more severe, and there may be a higher chance of needing prolonged medical care, even if they survive the initial infection.

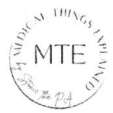

Factors Affecting Recovery for All Types of Pneumonia

Age: Older adults and young children may take longer to recover and are at higher risk for complications.

Pre-existing conditions: Chronic health conditions like asthma, COPD, heart disease, or diabetes can extend recovery time.

Treatment response: How well the patient responds to treatment (e.g., antibiotics, antivirals) and whether the pneumonia is caused by resistant bacteria or a virus can influence recovery time.

Summary

Mild pneumonia typically resolves in a few weeks with proper treatment, and full recovery is usually expected.

Severe pneumonia may require hospitalization and recovery could take weeks or even months, especially if complications arise.

Immunocompromised pneumonia can have a more unpredictable and prolonged recovery, as the body's ability to fight the infection is weakened.

For all types of pneumonia, follow-up care, good nutrition, rest, and sometimes rehabilitation are important parts of the recovery process.

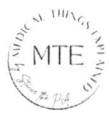

Sources:

Centers for Disease Control and Prevention (CDC):
CDC - Pneumonia

American Lung Association (ALA): ALA - Pneumonia

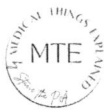

What is Pulmonary Rehab? Is Physical therapy needed?

Yes, **physical therapy** and **pulmonary rehabilitation** are often recommended after pneumonia, especially in cases of severe pneumonia or for individuals with underlying health conditions. These therapies help improve lung health, increase strength, and reduce the risk of long-term complications. Here's how they work:

1. Pulmonary Rehabilitation

Pulmonary rehabilitation is a specialized program designed to help people with respiratory conditions, including those recovering from pneumonia, improve lung function and overall health.

What It Involves:

Breathing Exercises: Techniques like diaphragmatic (belly) breathing and pursed-lip breathing help improve the efficiency of your breathing and reduce shortness of breath.

Physical Exercise: A structured exercise program helps strengthen the muscles used in breathing and improves overall endurance. Exercise can include walking, stationary biking, or other low-impact activities tailored to the individual's fitness level.

Education: Patients learn about lung health, how to manage their condition, and how to avoid triggers that can worsen breathing problems.

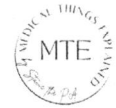

Nutritional Support: Diet and nutrition advice is also provided, as good nutrition is essential for recovery and overall lung health.

Why It's Beneficial:

After pneumonia, people may experience reduced lung capacity, shortness of breath, or weakness due to prolonged bed rest. Pulmonary rehab helps restore strength, improve oxygenation, and increase exercise tolerance, helping individuals return to normal activities.

It can also reduce hospital readmissions for those with pneumonia and other lung diseases like chronic obstructive pulmonary disease (COPD).

2. Physical Therapy

Physical therapy may also be used after pneumonia, particularly in cases where the patient has been hospitalized or has had extended bed rest. Physical therapists work with patients to improve overall physical strength and mobility.

What It Involves:

Strengthening Exercises: These exercises are aimed at rebuilding muscle strength, especially if the person has experienced muscle weakness due to being bedridden or using a ventilator.

Mobility Training: Some patients may need help with regaining balance and coordination. Therapists may guide them through walking exercises and teach safe techniques for getting out of bed or sitting up.

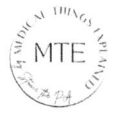

Postural Exercises: Helping the patient regain proper posture can reduce strain on the lungs and improve overall breathing.

Why It's Beneficial:

Regaining Strength: Pneumonia and prolonged hospitalization can lead to muscle weakness, and physical therapy helps the patient rebuild strength and stamina.

Improving Function: Physical therapy helps patients return to normal activities and maintain independence, especially for older adults or those with chronic health conditions.

Preventing Complications: Physical therapy can help prevent complications like blood clots (due to immobility) and improve overall mobility.

3. How Long Does It Take?

The duration of pulmonary rehabilitation or physical therapy varies depending on the severity of pneumonia, the patient's age, and their overall health.

For most people recovering from mild pneumonia, therapy may not be necessary, but for severe cases or patients with underlying conditions, therapy may last **several weeks to months** after hospitalization.

Many patients may start seeing benefits within the first few weeks, with continued improvements over time.

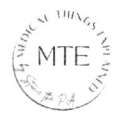

4. Who Needs Pulmonary Rehab or Physical Therapy After Pneumonia?

People with Severe Pneumonia: Those who have been hospitalized or had severe pneumonia may benefit the most from pulmonary rehabilitation and physical therapy.

Older Adults: Seniors often need rehabilitation because they may experience longer recovery times due to age-related factors.

People with Underlying Conditions: Individuals with conditions like asthma, COPD, or heart disease may need extra help in recovering from pneumonia and restoring their lung health.

Summary

After pneumonia, **pulmonary rehabilitation** and **physical therapy** can significantly aid in recovery by improving lung function, muscle strength, and overall physical endurance. These therapies are especially helpful for those who had severe pneumonia, were hospitalized, or have chronic health conditions. These programs are customized to each individual and can help speed up recovery, reduce the risk of future infections, and improve quality of life.

Sources:

American Lung Association (ALA): Pulmonary Rehabilitation

National Institutes of Health (NIH): Pulmonary Rehabilitation

Date: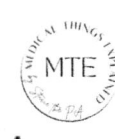

Quote Of The Day
_____
_____

Today I am truly grateful for...
_____
_____
_____
_____

Here's what would make today great...
_____
_____
_____
_____

I am...
_____
_____
_____

Some amazing things that happened today...
_____
_____

Some amazing things that happened today...
_____
_____

What could I have done to make today even better?
_____
_____

Date: _____

Quote Of The Day
_____
_____
_____

Today I am truly grateful for...
_____
_____
_____
_____
_____

Here's what would make today great...
_____
_____
_____
_____
_____

I am...
_____
_____
_____

Some amazing things that happened today...
_____
_____

Some amazing things that happened today...
_____
_____

What could I have done to make today even better?
_____
_____

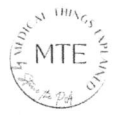

What is Mindfulness?

How do you do those exercises to reduce anxiety?

Mindfulness practices can be helpful during the recovery process from pneumonia, especially in managing stress, anxiety, and the discomfort that can come with breathing difficulties. Mindfulness involves focusing on the present moment and being aware of your thoughts, feelings, and bodily sensations without judgment. These practices can help reduce anxiety, improve breathing, and promote relaxation, which may enhance recovery and overall well-being.

Here are **five mindfulness exercises** that can be used in the setting of pneumonia recovery:

1. Mindful Breathing

How to do it: Sit or lie down in a comfortable position. Focus your attention on your breath, feeling the air as it enters and exits your body. If your mind begins to wander, gently bring it back to your breath. You can count your breaths (inhale for a count of 4, hold for 4, exhale for 4) to help focus your attention.

Why it helps: Mindful breathing promotes relaxation, helps reduce anxiety, and encourages deeper, slower breathing, which is essential for patients recovering from pneumonia. It can also help improve lung function and ease the feeling of breathlessness.

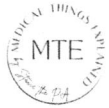

2. Body Scan Meditation

How to do it: Lie down in a comfortable position with your eyes closed. Begin by focusing your attention on your feet, noticing any sensations you feel there. Slowly move your focus upward, part by part—legs, abdomen, chest, arms, and head—while noticing any areas of tension or discomfort. Breathe into those areas and allow the tension to release with each exhale.

Why it helps: This exercise promotes body awareness, encourages relaxation, and helps release physical tension. For someone recovering from pneumonia, it can help relieve discomfort in the chest and ribs and reduce stress in the body.

3. Guided Visualization

How to do it: Close your eyes and take a few deep breaths. Imagine a peaceful, healing place, such as a quiet beach, a calm forest, or a gentle meadow. Picture the sights, sounds, and smells of this place. Imagine your lungs healing with each breath you take, filling your body with clean, fresh air.

Why it helps: Guided visualization can reduce anxiety, improve mood, and foster a positive mindset. It also encourages the patient to focus on healing and well-being, which can be especially beneficial during the recovery process from pneumonia.

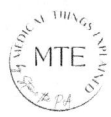

4. Mindful Movement (Gentle Stretching or Yoga)

How to do it: Perform simple, slow stretches or gentle yoga poses while focusing on your breath and bodily sensations. Focus on moving slowly and mindfully, paying attention to how each movement feels in your body. Make sure not to push your body too hard—gentle movements are key.

Why it helps: Gentle stretching or yoga can help improve circulation, relieve chest tightness, and promote lung expansion. Mindfully moving the body can also help reduce stress and muscle stiffness, which can occur when recovering from pneumonia.

5. Loving-Kindness Meditation (Metta)

How to do it: Sit comfortably with your eyes closed and take a few deep breaths. Focus on sending feelings of warmth, love, and compassion to yourself first, saying silently, "May I be safe, may I be healthy, may I be happy, may I live with ease." Then, gradually extend these wishes to others—family members, friends, or even people you don't know.

Why it helps: Loving-kindness meditation helps reduce negative emotions like anxiety or fear and promotes feelings of connection and compassion. It can help patients feel more at ease during their recovery, supporting both emotional and physical healing.

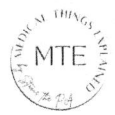

Benefits of Mindfulness Practices for Pneumonia Recovery

Reduces Stress: Mindfulness helps calm the nervous system, reducing anxiety about the illness or recovery process, which can in turn improve overall health.

Improves Breathing: Mindful breathing exercises can promote more efficient lung function and improve oxygen intake, especially when recovering from pneumonia.

Promotes Relaxation: Mindfulness encourages relaxation, which can help manage pain and discomfort associated with pneumonia recovery.

Fosters Positive Thinking: Practices like loving-kindness meditation and visualization help shift focus from negative thoughts or fear to healing and well-being.

Improves Sleep: Mindfulness can help improve sleep quality by reducing anxiety and promoting relaxation, which is important for recovery.

In Summary:

Mindfulness exercises are simple, accessible tools that can support physical and emotional healing during pneumonia recovery. These practices help patients focus on their breath, reduce stress, and promote relaxation, ultimately contributing to faster recovery and a more positive outlook.

SECTION 7
Impact on Relationships and Self-Image

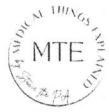

How Pneumonia Affects Spouses and Family Members

1. **Emotional Stress**

Fear and Anxiety: The sudden onset of pneumonia, especially if it leads to hospitalization or severe symptoms, can cause anxiety and fear. Family members may worry about the loved one's health, the possibility of complications, or even death, especially in older adults or those with pre-existing conditions.

Uncertainty: Pneumonia recovery can take time, and the course of the illness can be unpredictable. This uncertainty can cause stress and worry for the spouse or family members, who may not know how long recovery will take or what complications might arise.

2. **Physical and Mental Fatigue**

Caregiving responsibilities: A spouse or family member may take on the role of primary caregiver, helping with tasks like cooking, cleaning, managing medications, or providing transportation to doctor's appointments. This added responsibility can be exhausting, both physically and mentally.

Sleep Disruptions: Caring for a sick loved one, particularly one with breathing difficulties or who needs frequent medical attention, can disrupt the family's sleep routine. Lack of rest can lead to fatigue, affecting the ability to manage daily tasks and emotional well-being.

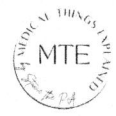

3. Role Changes and Family Dynamics

Shifts in daily roles: Family roles may shift when someone is hospitalized or bedridden due to pneumonia. The primary caregiver may have to take on new responsibilities, such as managing finances, childcare, or household chores, while also supporting the patient emotionally.

Financial strain: If the person with pneumonia cannot work for an extended period or if hospitalization is required, the family may face financial challenges. Medical bills and missed income can add stress to the situation, making it difficult for family members to focus on recovery.

4. Impact on Children

Fear and confusion: Children may struggle to understand why their parent or caregiver is suddenly very sick, especially if pneumonia leads to hospitalization. Young children may experience fear, confusion, or anxiety about the illness, and older children might take on more household duties, affecting their routine and school performance.

Stress and Adjustment: Children might feel emotionally burdened by the changes in family dynamics or the emotional stress of seeing a loved one so ill. They may worry about the potential loss of the person who is ill or have difficulty coping with the change in family roles.

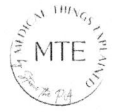

Understanding the Emotional Impact on Loved Ones

1. Feelings of Helplessness

Family members and spouses may feel **helpless** when a loved one is struggling with pneumonia. The illness can cause extreme weakness, difficulty breathing, and pain, and loved ones may feel powerless in the face of the patient's distress. This feeling of helplessness can be overwhelming, particularly when they cannot make their loved one feel better quickly.

2. Guilt and Self-Blame

Family members may feel **guilty** about not noticing symptoms sooner or worry that they could have done something to prevent the illness. In some cases, they may feel responsible for not managing the person's health properly or for exposing them to the illness in the first place, even though many cases of pneumonia are not preventable.

3. Emotional Burnout

Caregiving can be physically and emotionally draining, and family members may experience **caregiver burnout**. This can lead to feelings of frustration, isolation, or resentment, especially if they feel they have to do everything themselves. Burnout can also result from emotional exhaustion caused by worry, fear, and watching a loved one suffer.

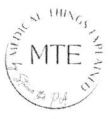

4. Depression and Anxiety

The stress and emotional toll of caring for someone with pneumonia can increase the risk of **depression** and **anxiety** among family members. Anxiety about the patient's recovery, especially if the illness becomes severe, can result in sleepless nights, irritability, or constant worry. Spouses may also feel **lonely** or disconnected if they cannot spend time together as they used to due to the illness.

How Families Can Cope with the Emotional Impact of Pneumonia

1. Communication and Support

Open communication is key to reducing stress. Family members should encourage each other to talk about their feelings and worries. **Sharing responsibilities** and staying connected can ease the emotional burden.

Support groups or **counseling** can help family members cope with the emotional impact of the illness. Having a space to talk with others who are experiencing similar challenges can provide comfort and a sense of solidarity.

2. Self-Care for Caregivers

Family members and caregivers must also take time to care for themselves. This might mean asking for help from other family members or friends, taking breaks, or finding moments of relaxation to recharge. Maintaining their own physical and mental health is crucial to being able to provide effective care for their loved one.

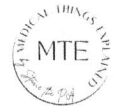

Mindfulness practices, **exercise**, and **relaxation techniques** can help caregivers manage stress and avoid burnout.

3. **Seeking Professional Help**

If emotional stress becomes overwhelming, seeking help from a mental health professional can be beneficial. A therapist or counselor can help family members navigate feelings of anxiety, guilt, or depression.

Medical providers can also offer resources for emotional support, such as recommending support groups, counseling, or connecting families to community resources.

4. **Encouraging Patient Participation**

For the patient recovering from pneumonia, involving them in decisions about their recovery can reduce feelings of helplessness. Encouraging them to set small, achievable goals for recovery, such as walking short distances or participating in light activities, can empower them and help family members feel more hopeful about the recovery process.

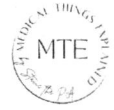

How does an illness like pneumonia affect intimacy and self esteem?

Pneumonia and its recovery can have an impact on a person's sex life and self-image, particularly if the illness was severe or required hospitalization. The physical, emotional, and psychological effects of the illness can contribute to changes in how a person feels about themselves and their body, as well as how they relate to their partner in an intimate way.

1. Effects on Sex Life During Pneumonia Recovery

Physical Exhaustion and Weakness

> **Fatigue** is a common symptom of pneumonia recovery, especially in severe cases or for those who were hospitalized. The body requires significant energy to fight the infection, and after weeks of illness or treatment, a person may feel physically drained.
>
> **Breathing difficulties**: Pneumonia often affects the lungs, causing shortness of breath or difficulty breathing, which can make physical activity, including sex, more challenging or uncomfortable. This can reduce sexual desire or enjoyment.
>
> **Muscle weakness**: If a person spent time in bed or was on a ventilator, they may experience muscle weakness, which can affect stamina and the ability to engage in physical intimacy comfortably.

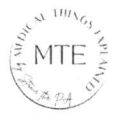

Impact of Medication

> Some medications used to treat pneumonia, such as **antibiotics** or **pain relievers**, can affect libido or cause temporary side effects like **nausea, fatigue,** or **dizziness,** making the thought of sex less appealing.
>
> In addition, certain medications, especially steroids or sedatives, may affect hormone levels, which could contribute to a decrease in sexual desire.

Emotional and Psychological Effects

> **Anxiety and Stress**: Recovering from a serious illness like pneumonia can cause feelings of **anxiety** or **depression**, which can affect a person's mental state and reduce their interest in intimacy.
>
> **Fear of Re-infection or Complications**: Some individuals may feel **fearful** about resuming physical intimacy because they're concerned about their body's ability to handle the strain or about the possibility of re-infection.
>
> **Loss of Self-Confidence**: If pneumonia has caused a significant physical toll, such as weight loss, muscle atrophy, or changes in appearance due to prolonged bed rest, a person might feel self-conscious or embarrassed, affecting their sexual confidence.

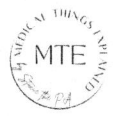

2. Effects on Self-Image During Pneumonia Recovery

Changes in Body Image

> **Physical appearance:** After pneumonia, especially if hospitalization was involved, a person may have lost weight or muscle mass due to illness or inactivity. They may feel weaker, fatigued, or not like the way their body looks, which can affect their **self-esteem** and **body image**.
>
> **Breathing difficulties**: If a person had severe pneumonia, they might still feel short of breath or tired, even after recovery, which can make them feel less physically capable or self-conscious.
>
> **Scarring or medical equipment marks**: If a person was intubated, had a chest tube, or received other invasive treatments, there may be visible scars or marks that can affect how they perceive their body.

Mental and Emotional Health

> **Depression**: Being bedridden or unable to engage in normal daily activities due to pneumonia can affect a person's mood, leading to depression. Depression, in turn, can contribute to a lower self-image and reduced desire for intimacy.

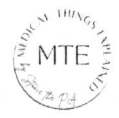

Sense of vulnerability: Illness can lead to feelings of vulnerability and helplessness, which may affect how a person perceives themselves in the context of their relationships. This can cause anxiety or self-doubt, especially about physical or emotional intimacy with a partner.

3. How to Address the Impact on Sex Life and Self-Image

For the Person Recovering from Pneumonia:

Allow time for recovery: It's important to give the body time to heal physically and emotionally. Trying to return to sexual activity too soon may cause stress or exhaustion.

Communicate with your partner: Talking openly with your partner about feelings, physical limitations, and any fears related to sex and intimacy can help both partners understand each other's needs and reduce anxiety.

Gentle intimacy: Resuming intimacy doesn't have to mean jumping back into full sexual activity. It can start with **gentle touch, cuddling,** or **holding hands**—any form of intimacy that feels comfortable.

Focus on self-care: Taking care of your mental and physical health—whether through rest, nutrition, relaxation, or seeking counseling—can help improve self-esteem and the ability to engage in intimacy when ready.

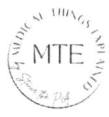

For Partners:

> **Patience and empathy**: If your partner is recovering from pneumonia, it's important to offer **patience**, understanding, and emotional support. Don't pressure them into intimacy before they're ready.
>
> **Encourage self-esteem**: Compliment your partner and express love and appreciation for who they are, not just their physical appearance, to help boost their confidence.
>
> **Physical closeness**: Engage in **non-sexual forms of physical closeness** like touching, massaging, or holding hands, which can help maintain the emotional bond without the pressure of sexual activity.

4. Seeking Professional Help

> If emotional or physical issues persist, such as **depression**, **anxiety**, or **relationship strain** due to the illness, it may be helpful to consult a healthcare provider or a **therapist**. Counseling can help manage mental health issues, rebuild self-esteem, and improve intimacy in relationships.

Summary

Pneumonia can affect a person's **sex life** and **self-image** due to physical exhaustion, changes in body appearance, emotional stress, and the impact of medications. It can also impact how they view themselves and their ability to engage in intimate relationships. Open communication, patience, and allowing time for both physical and emotional recovery are key to managing the effects of pneumonia on intimacy and self-image.

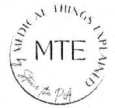

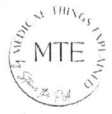

SECTION 8

Resources and References

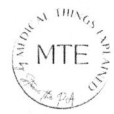

Resources and References

The information provided is based on general guidelines and recommendations from well-known health organizations, such as:

American Lung Association (ALA): The ALA provides guidelines on pneumonia symptoms, diagnosis, and treatment, with specific emphasis on prevention strategies such as vaccination and smoking cessation. American Lung Association - Pneumonia, Pulmonary Rehabilitation

American Thoracic Society (ATS): Offers in-depth information about pleural decortication, its indications, and the role of thoracic surgeons. ATS - Pleural Disease

Centers for Disease Control and Prevention (CDC): The CDC offers detailed information on the diagnosis, treatment, and prevention of pneumonia. Their guidelines include information for both bacterial and viral pneumonia, as well as specific considerations for severe and immunocompromised patients. CDC - Pneumonia

National Institutes of Health (NIH): The NIH provides extensive resources on respiratory health, including pneumonia diagnosis, treatment options, and care for vulnerable populations like those with weakened immune systems. NIH - Pneumonia, Pulmonary Rehabilitation

National Institute for Health and Care Excellence (NICE): Provides guidelines for managing complications of pneumonia, including pleural effusion and empyema. NICE - Pleural Disease

SECTION 9

Medical Summary

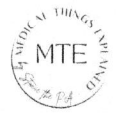

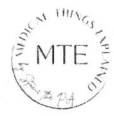

Personal Medical Summary:

Personal Information:

Full Name:
_____

Date of Birth: _____

Blood Type: _____

Drug Allergies: _____

Emergency Contacts:

Name: _____

Relationship: _____

Phone: _____

Name: _____

Relationship: _____

Phone: _____

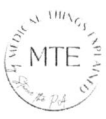

Power of Attorney or Health Care Surrogate:

Name: _____

Relationship: _____

Phone: _____

Name: _____

Relationship: _____

Phone: _____

Notes:

_____

_____

_____

_____

_____

_____

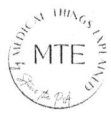

Medical Conditions / Diagnosis

- _____
- _____
- _____
- _____
- _____
- _____
- _____
- _____
- _____
- _____
- _____
- _____

Circle if you have: alcohol or substance abuse, arrhythmias, chronic pain medications, COPD (Chronic Obstructive Pulmonary Disease), diabetes, heart failure, hemophilia, kidney disease, liver disease, psychiatric disorders, seizures, stroke, TIA (Transient Ischemic Attack)

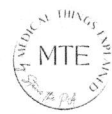

Medications/Devices:

Name	Dose	How often	Reason/MD

Circle if you use: AICD, AV fistula, BiPAP, bladder stimulator, cane, cochlear implants, CPAP, dentures/partials, hearing aids, insulin pump, intrathecal pain pump, oxygen, pacemaker, peritoneal catheter, prosthetic devices, spinal cord stimulator, urinary catheter, vagus nerve stimulator, walker, and wearable pain patches.

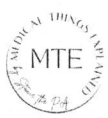

Allergies / Sensitivities

Medications/Reaction:
_____
_____
_____
_____
_____

Foods or Environmental:
_____
_____

Other:
_____
_____
_____
_____

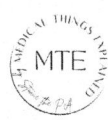

Surgeries / Procedures

Surgery: _____

Date/MD: _____

Surgery: _____

Date/MD: _____

Surgery: _____

Date/MD: _____

Circle if you had: Any heart surgery (such as bypass or valve replacement), bariatric surgery, brain surgery (like craniotomy), cesarean section or hysterectomy, gallbladder removal (cholecystectomy), joint replacement (hip, knee, shoulder), organ transplant, spinal surgery (like laminectomy or fusion), stent placement or angioplasty, and any recent abdominal surgery

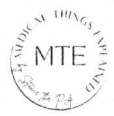

Recent Hospital Visits or Emergency Events

Reason: _____ Date: _____

Reason: _____ Date: _____

Reason: _____ Date: _____

Reason: _____ Date: _____

Reason: _____ Date: _____

Reason: _____ Date: _____

Reason: _____ Date: _____

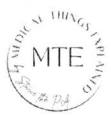

Family History (Relevant Medical Conditions)

- _____
- _____
- _____

Doctor Information:

Primary Care Provider: _____

Phone/Fax: _____

Cardiologist: _____

Phone/Fax: _____

Oncologist:_____

Phone/Fax: _____

Surgeon:_____

Phone/Fax: _____

Pulmonologist:_____

Phone/Fax: _____

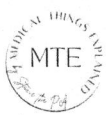

Insurance Information: copy cards and keep here

Insurance Provider: _____

Secondary Provider:_____

Additional Information (Optional)

Advanced Directives or DNR: (e.g., "Yes, copy on file with PCP")

Special Instructions:

_____

_____

Tips for Use

- Keep this summary in your **wallet** or **phone** in case of emergency.
- **Update regularly** with any new medications, surgeries, or diagnoses.
- Consider sharing a copy with **family members** or emergency contacts.

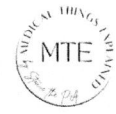

BLOOD PRESSURE LOG

Name. _____

Date	AM		PM		Notes
	Blood pressure	Pulse	Blood pressure	Pulse	

BLOOD PRESSURE CATEGORY	SYSTOLIC mm Hg (upper number)	and/or	DIASTOLIC mm Hg (lower number)
NORMAL BLOOD PRESSURE	LESS THAN 120	and	LESS THAN 80
ELEVATED	120 – 129	and	LESS THAN 80
HIGH BLOOD PRESSURE (HYPERTENSION) STAGE 1	130 – 139	or	80 – 89
HIGH BLOOD PRESSURE (HYPERTENSION) STAGE 2	140 OR HIGHER	or	90 OR HIGHER
HYPERTENSIVE CRISIS (consult your doctor immediately)	HIGHER THAN 180	and/or	HIGHER THAN 120

FOOD JOURNAL

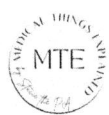

Breakfast   Servings   Calories

	Servings	Calories
		Subtotal

Snack

	Servings	Calories
		Subtotal

Lunch

	Servings	Calories
		Subtotal

Snack

	Servings	Calories
		Subtotal

Dinner

	Servings	Calories
		Subtotal

Snack

	Servings	Calories
		Subtotal

Total Calories From Food [ ]

FITNESS ACTIVITY JOURNAL

	Duration	Calories

Total Calories From Fitness [ ]

NOTES

FOOD JOURNAL

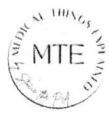

Breakfast   **Servings**   **Calories**

	Servings	Calories
		Subtotal

Snack

		Subtotal

Lunch

		Subtotal

Snack

		Subtotal

Dinner

		Subtotal

Snack

		Subtotal

Total Calories From Food [ ]

FITNESS ACTIVITY JOURNAL

	Duration	Calories

Total Calories From Fitness [ ]

NOTES

SECTION 10

Distracting Activities

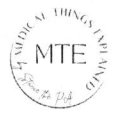

Maze #1

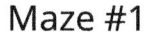

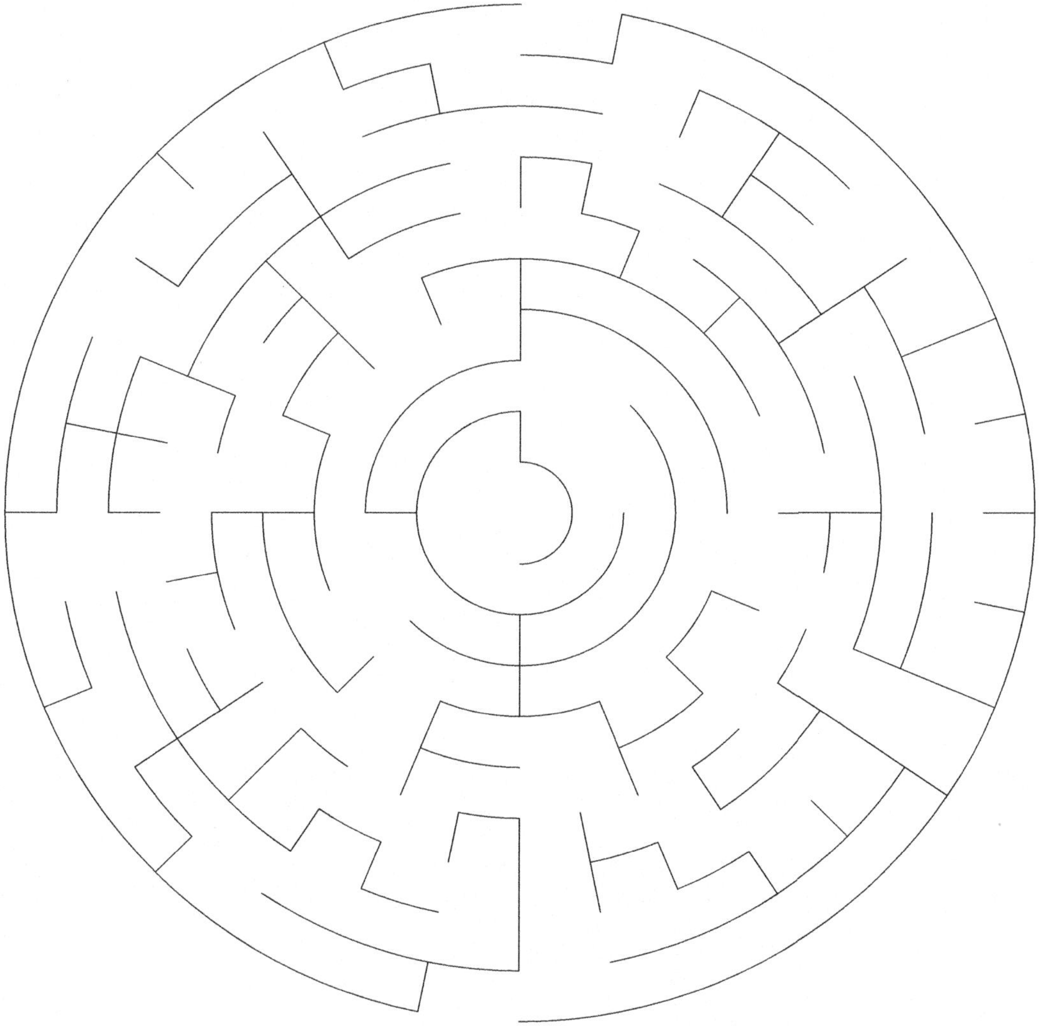

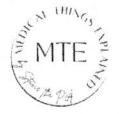

Maze #2

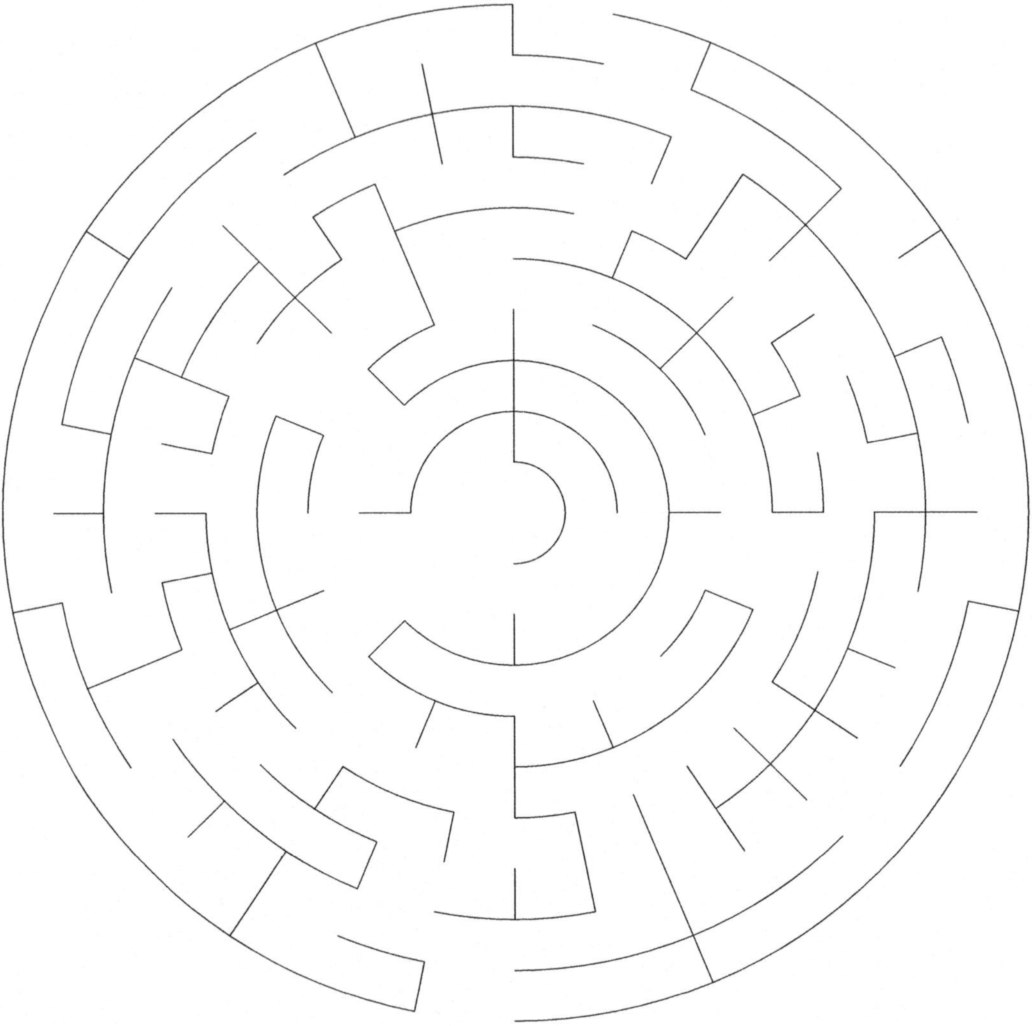

Maze #3

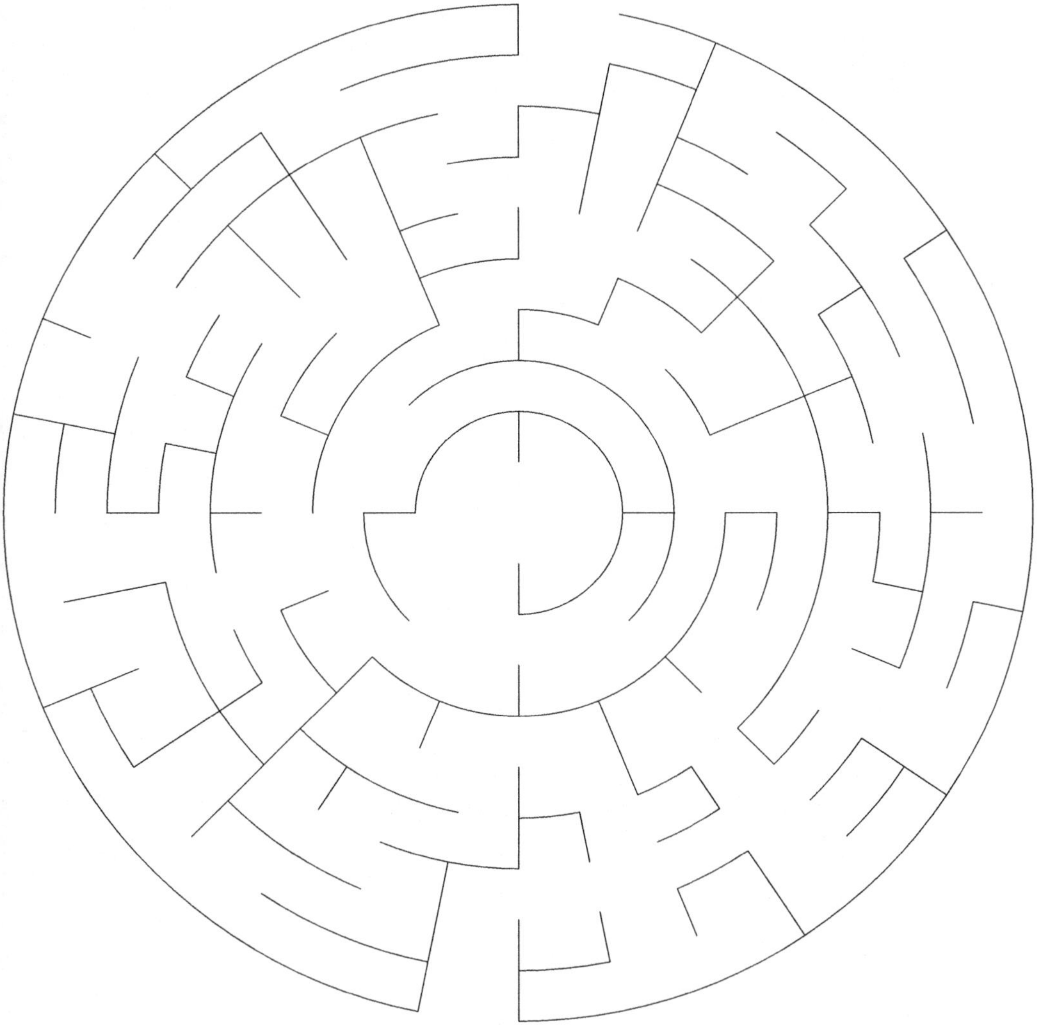

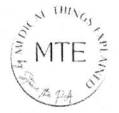

Maze #4

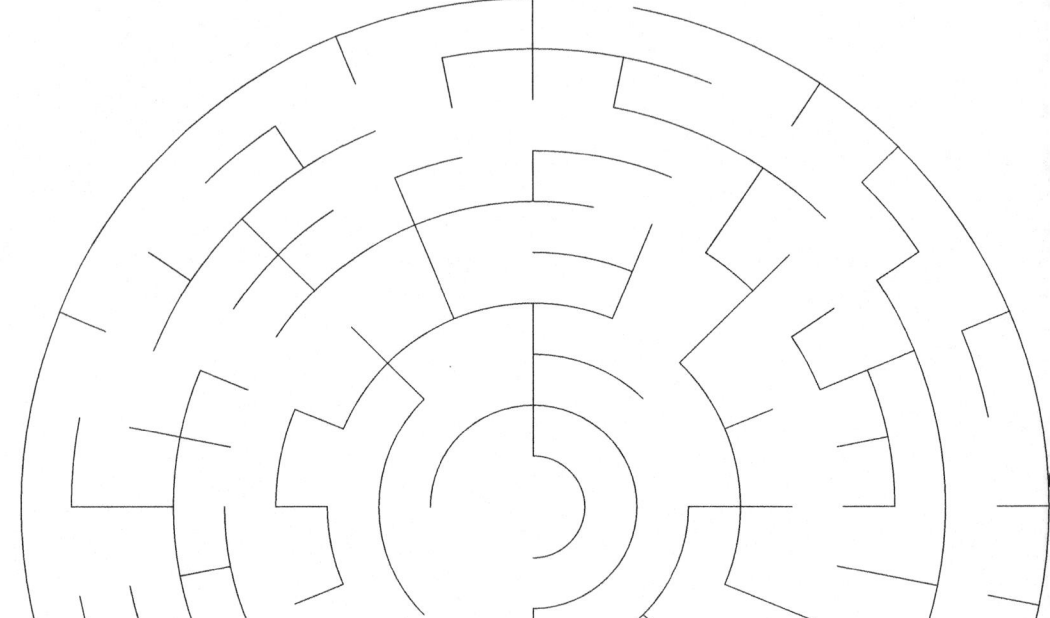

Maze Solution #1

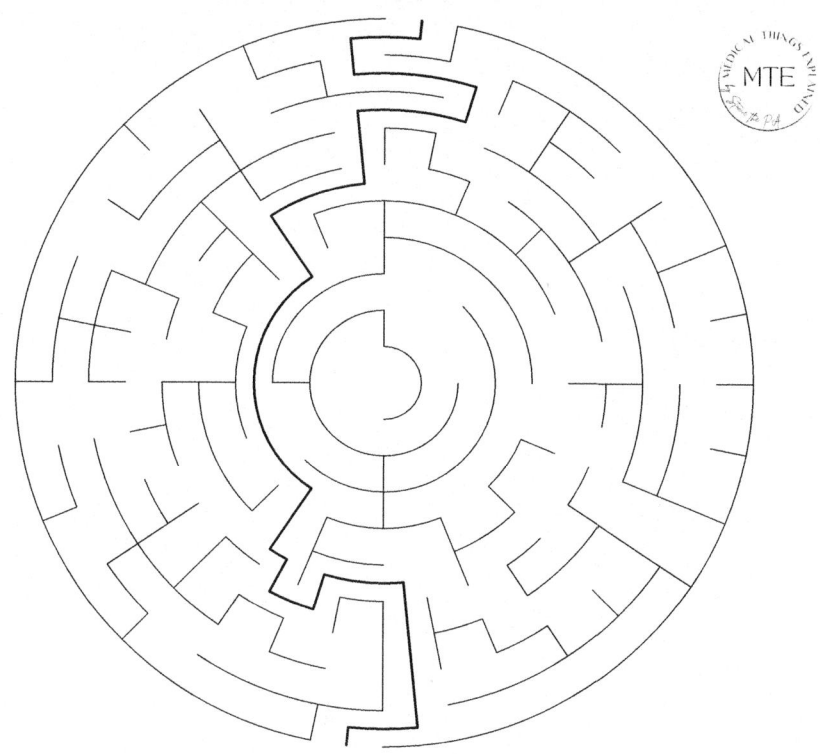

Maze Solution #2

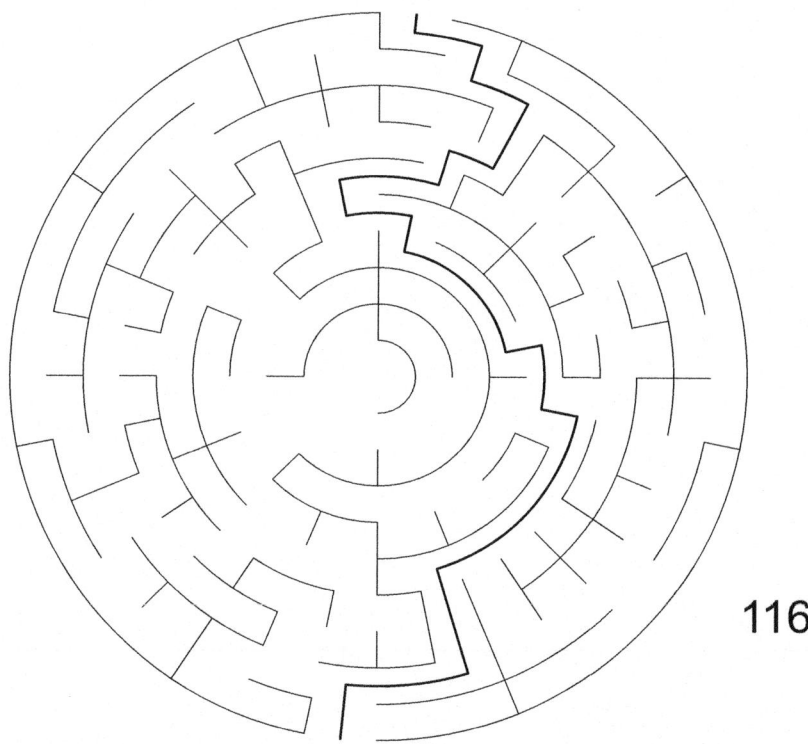

Maze Solution #3

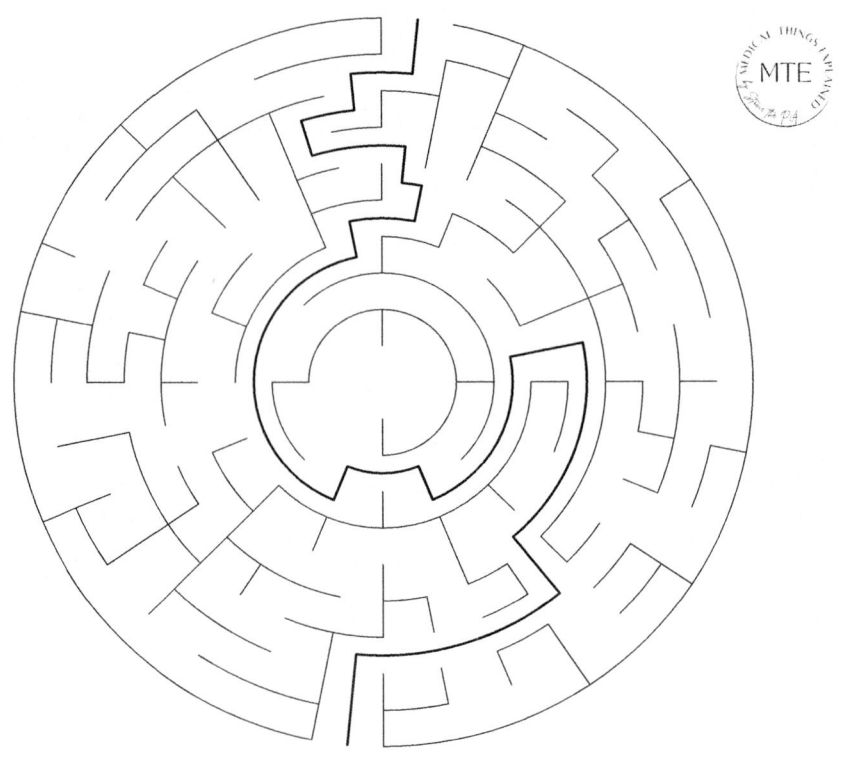

Maze Solution #4

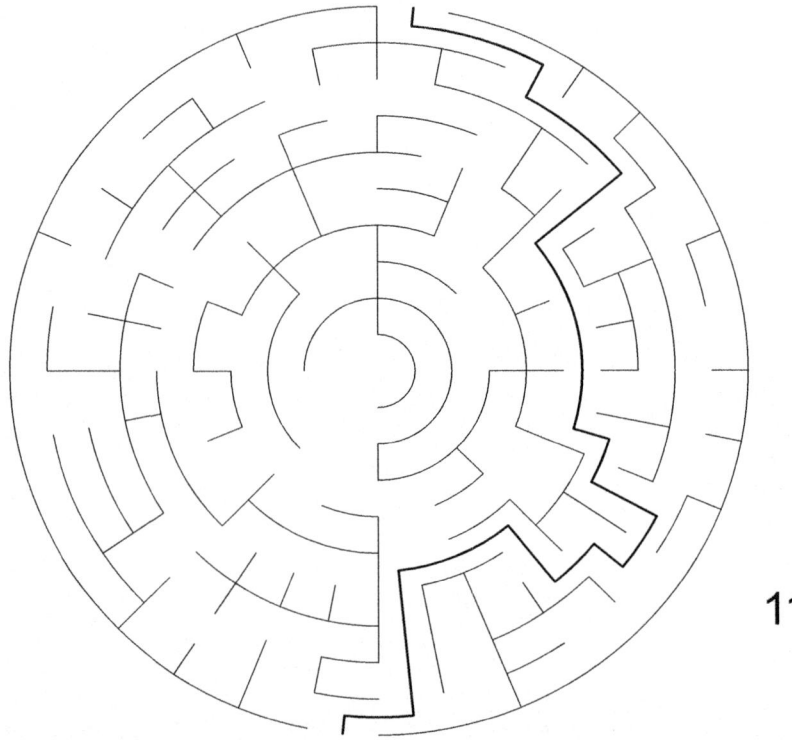

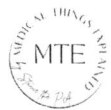

Disclaimer:
This workbook provides general information about pneumonia and related medical topics for educational purposes only. The content is not intended to diagnose, treat, or provide specific medical advice. It is not a substitute for professional medical judgment, diagnosis, or treatment. Always consult a licensed healthcare provider or physician for any medical concerns, symptoms, or questions. Do not disregard or delay seeking medical advice or treatment based on information found in this workbook. In the event of a medical emergency, immediately contact your healthcare provider or call 911 or your local emergency services.

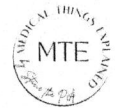

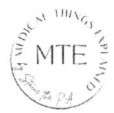

Thank you for choosing this workbook on pneumonia. Taking the time to understand your health is an important step in feeling more confident and less anxious about your condition. Knowledge is a powerful tool—it helps you manage symptoms, avoid future issues, and feel more in control of your well-being.

By learning more about your health, you're empowering yourself to make informed decisions, ask the right questions, and take the best possible care of yourself and your loved ones. This workbook is just one step on your health journey, and I encourage you to keep exploring other resources to continue building your knowledge and peace of mind.

Your health matters, and the more you know, the more you can live with confidence. Stay curious, stay proactive, and take charge of your health!

Stacie, PA-C

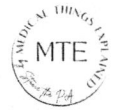

57 1975

Printed in Great Britain
by Amazon